Nana's Favorite Things

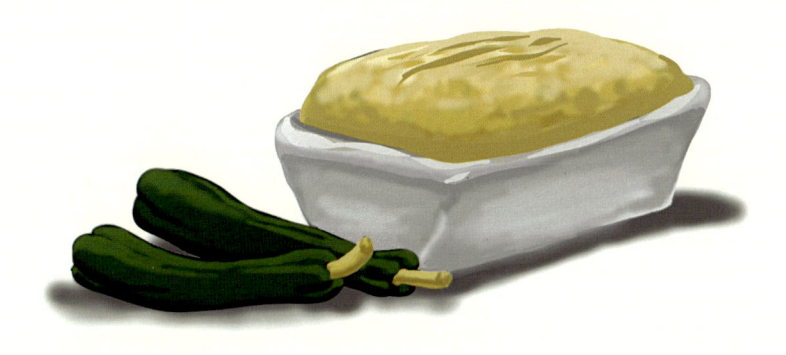

by Dorothy H. Price

illustrated by TeMika Grooms

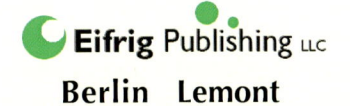

Eifrig Publishing LLC

Berlin   Lemont

© 2016 Dorothy H. Price
Printed in the United States of America

All rights reserved. This publication is protected by Copyright, and permission should be obtained from the publisher prior to any prohibited reproduction, storage in a retrieval system, or transmission in any form or by any means, electronic, mechanical, photocopying, recording, or likewise.

Published by Eifrig Publishing,
PO Box 66, Lemont, PA 16851, USA
Knobelsdorffstr. 44, 14059 Berlin, Germany.

For information regarding permission, write to:
Rights and Permissions Department,
Eifrig Publishing,
PO Box 66, Lemont, PA 16851, USA.
permissions@eifrigpublishing.com, +1-888-340-6543

Library of Congress Cataloging-in-Publication Data

Nana's Favorite Things
by Dorothy H. Price, illustrated by TeMika Grooms
p. cm.

Paperback: ISBN 978-1-63233-015-4
Hard cover: ISBN 978-1-63233-016-1

[1.Diabetes- Juvenile Fiction. 2. Healthy Living - Juvenile Fiction.]

I. Grooms, TeMika , ill. II. Title

20 19 18 17 2016
5 4 3 2 1
Printed on acid-free paper. ∞

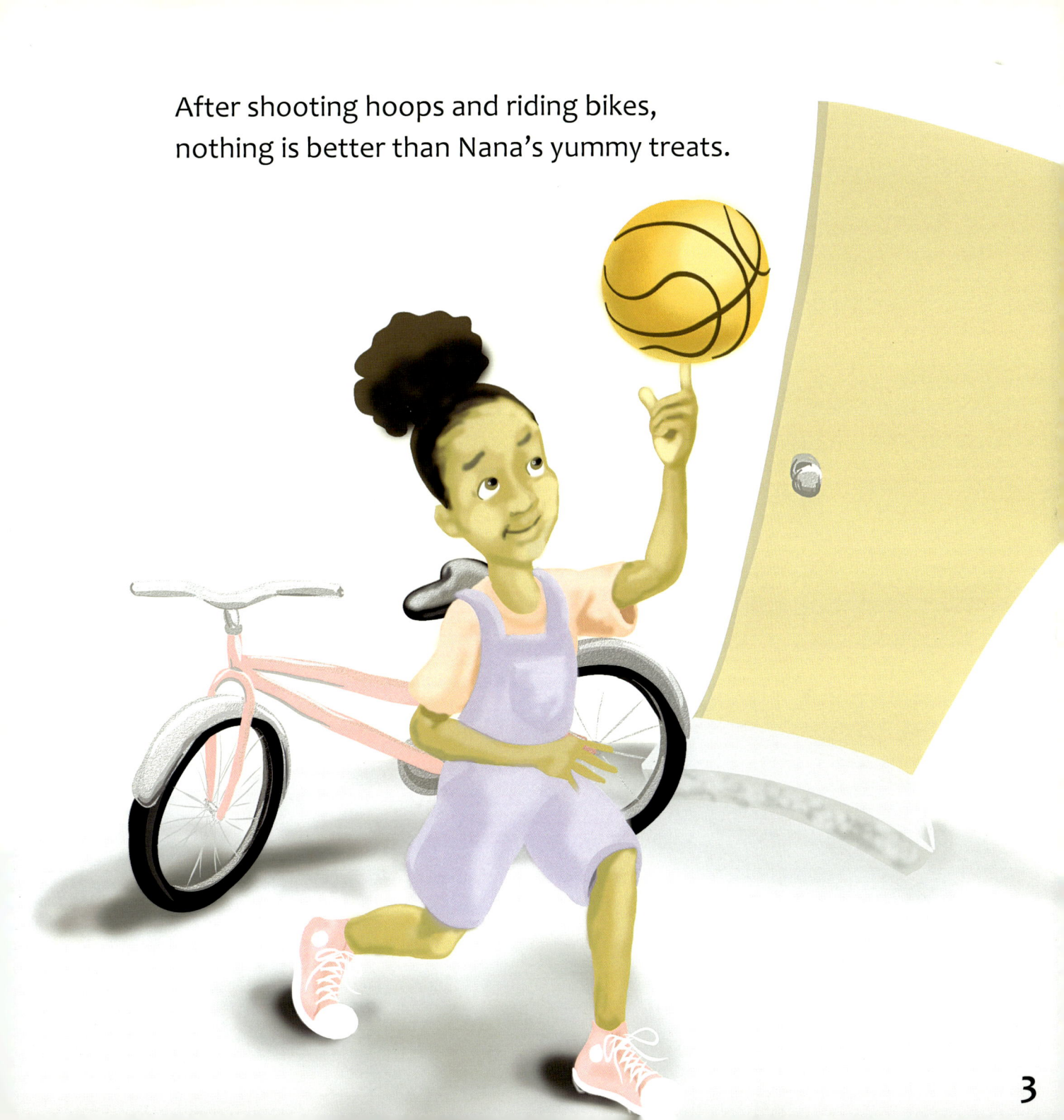

After shooting hoops and riding bikes, nothing is better than Nana's yummy treats.

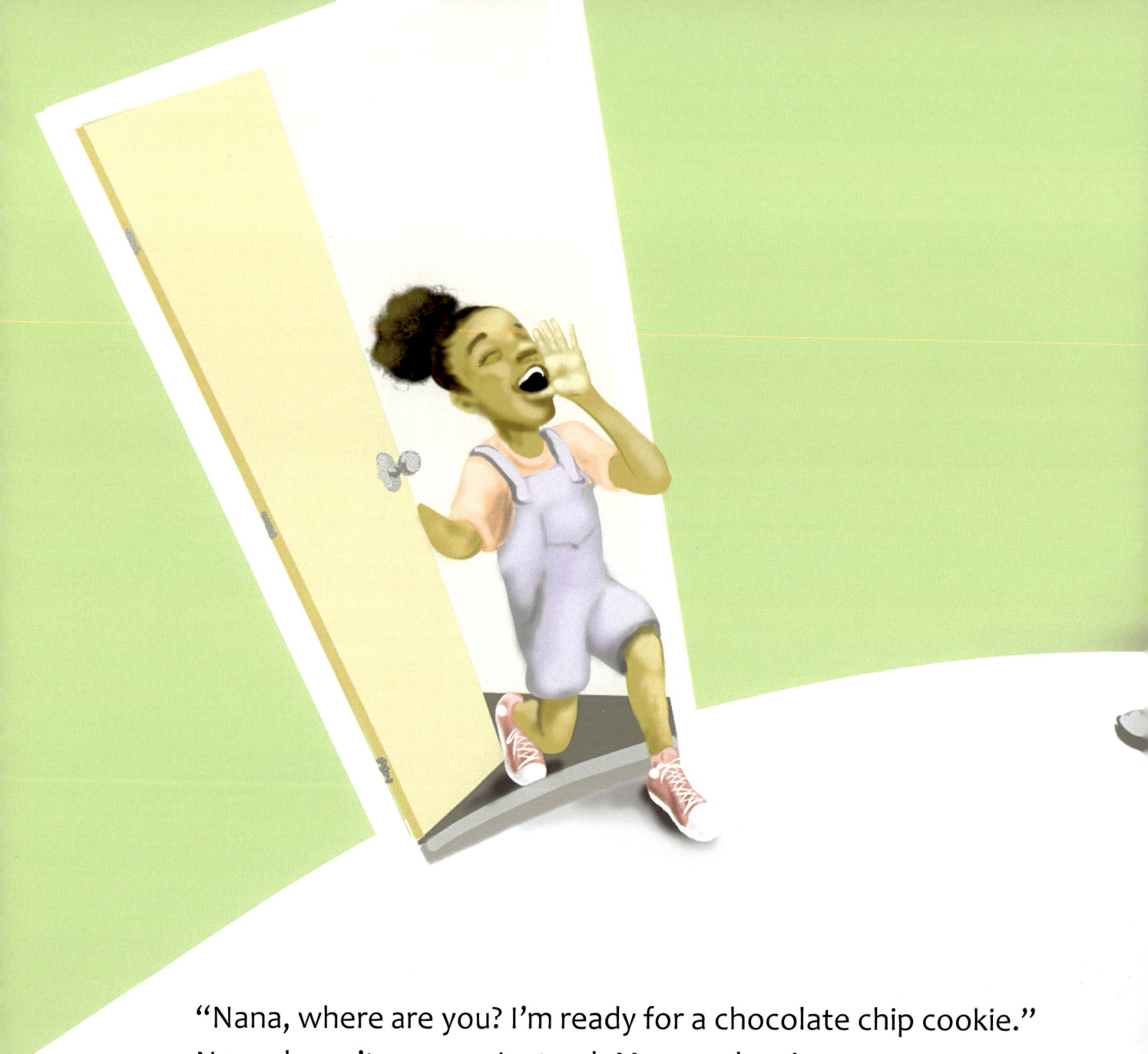

"Nana, where are you? I'm ready for a chocolate chip cookie."
Nana doesn't answer. Instead, Mom rushes in.
"Sasha, Nana isn't feeling well."

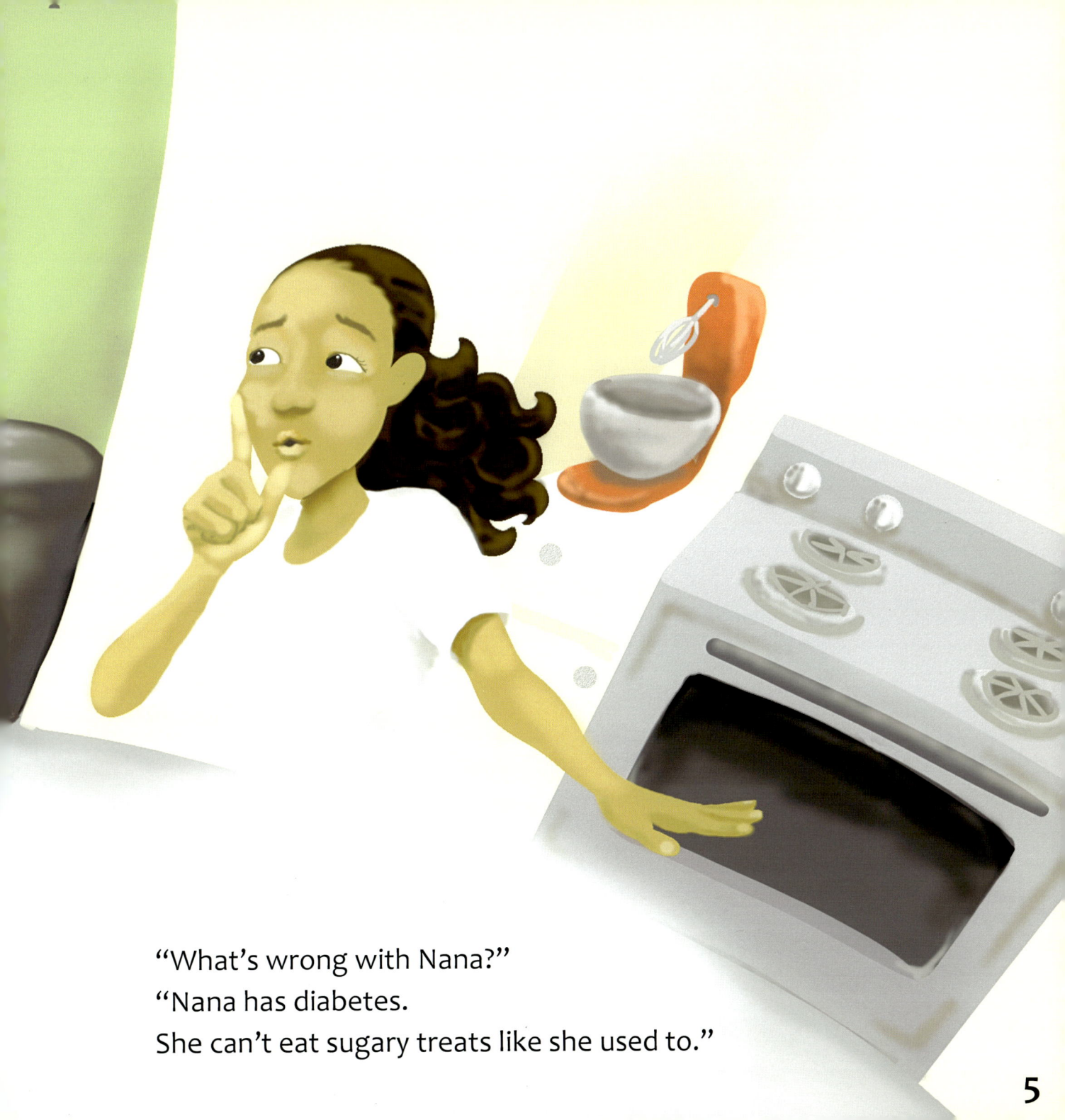

"What's wrong with Nana?"
"Nana has diabetes.
She can't eat sugary treats like she used to."

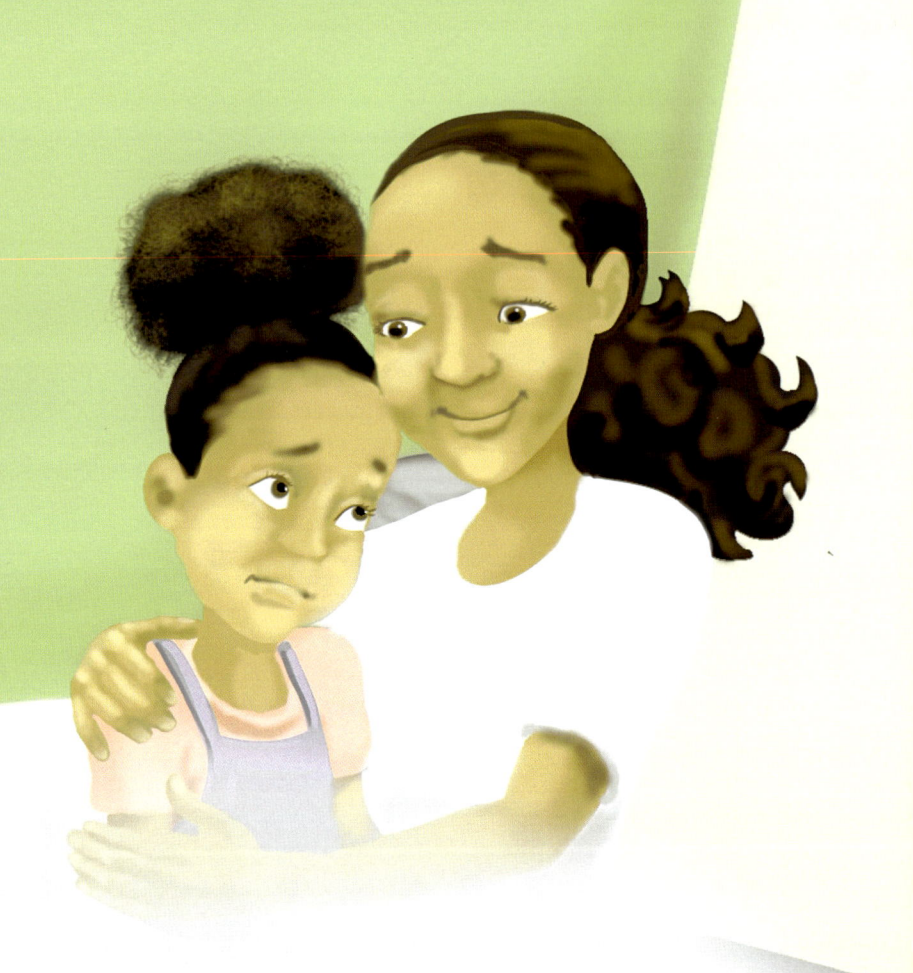

"Did I make Nana get diabetes by always asking for her cookies?"
"Of course not," Mom replied with a hug.
"Nana needs to exercise and eat healthier foods.
Then she'll be just fine."

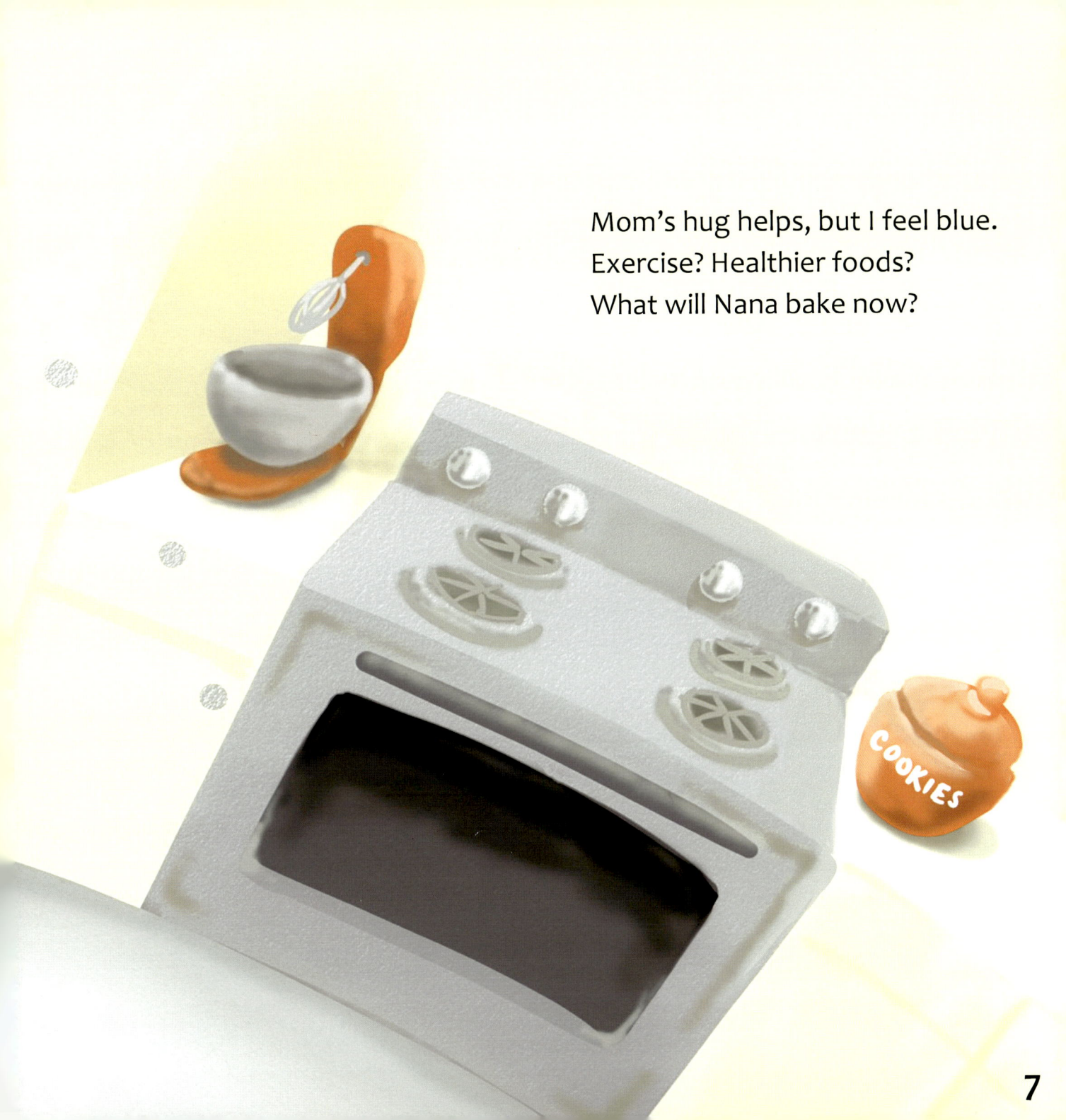

Mom's hug helps, but I feel blue.
Exercise? Healthier foods?
What will Nana bake now?

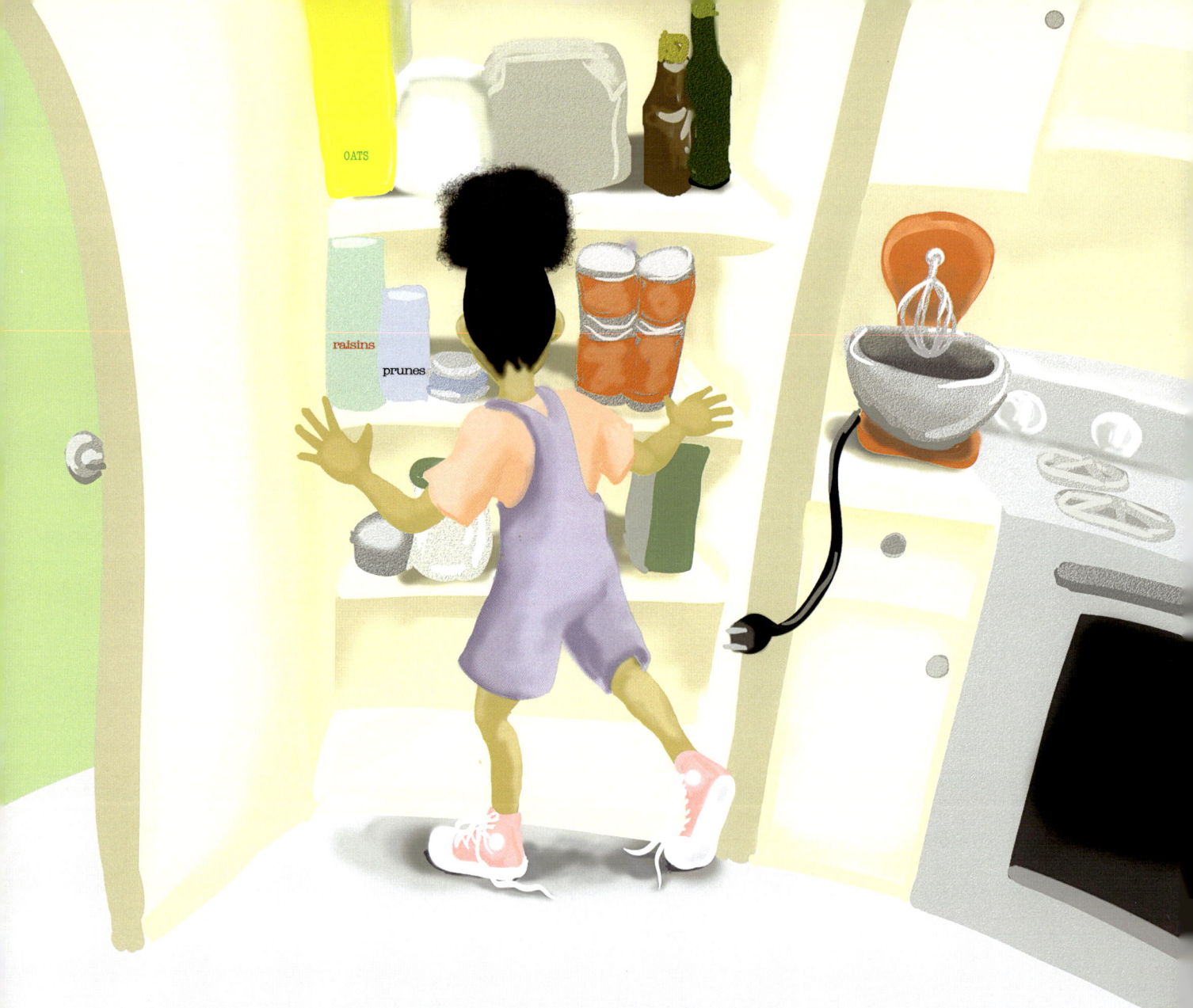

Walking into the pantry for a snack, I trip over my shiny shoelaces on my favorite pink high-tops, careful not to knock Nana's mixer onto the floor. She is always telling me to keep my laces tied, especially when I ride my bike.

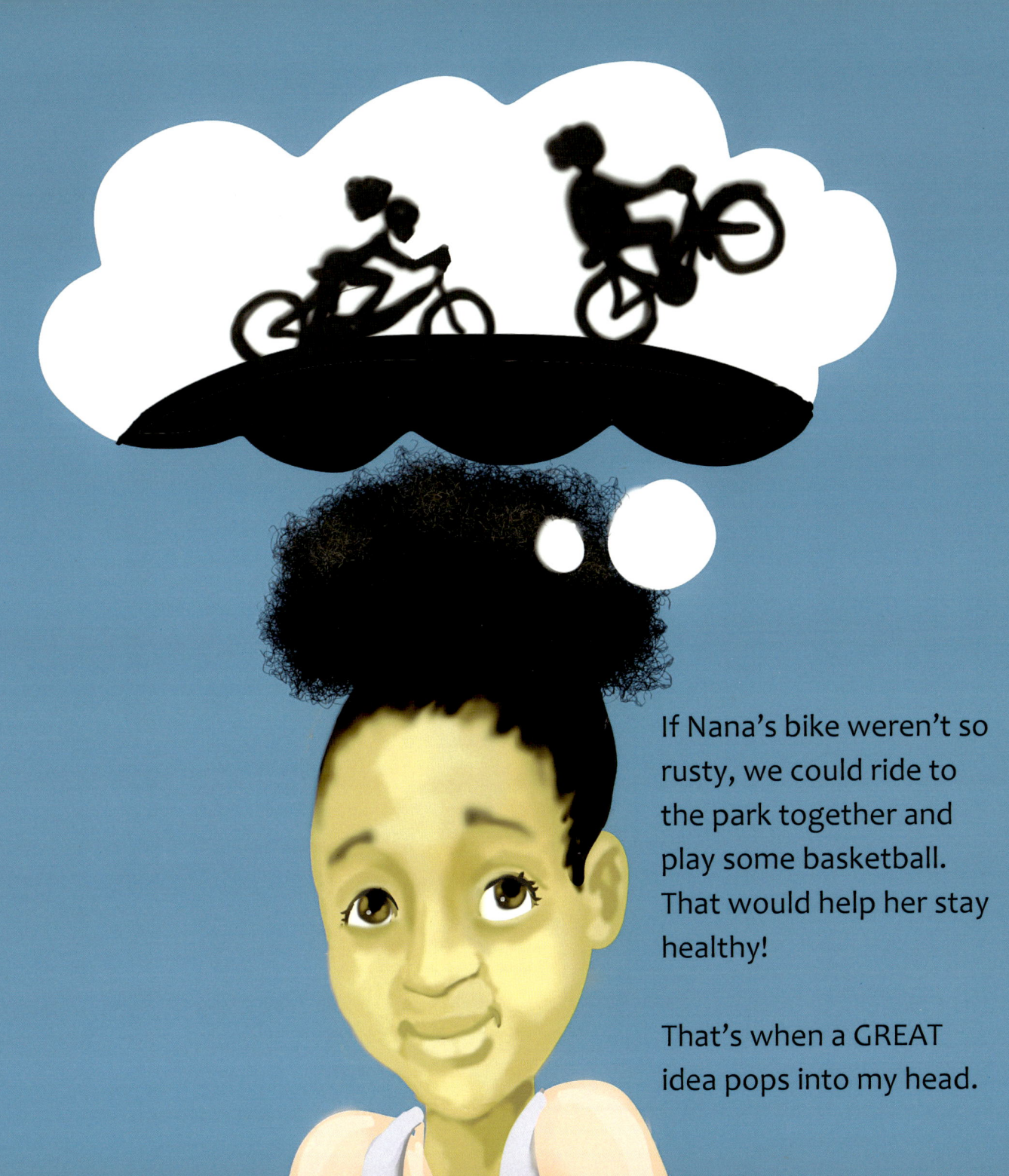

If Nana's bike weren't so rusty, we could ride to the park together and play some basketball. That would help her stay healthy!

That's when a GREAT idea pops into my head.

"I'll be right back," I tell Mom and race to my room.
I find my allowance and count how much I've saved for a new scooter. I would rather spend it on the perfect gift for Nana, but it's not quite enough. I'll have to empty my piggy bank, too. Got it!

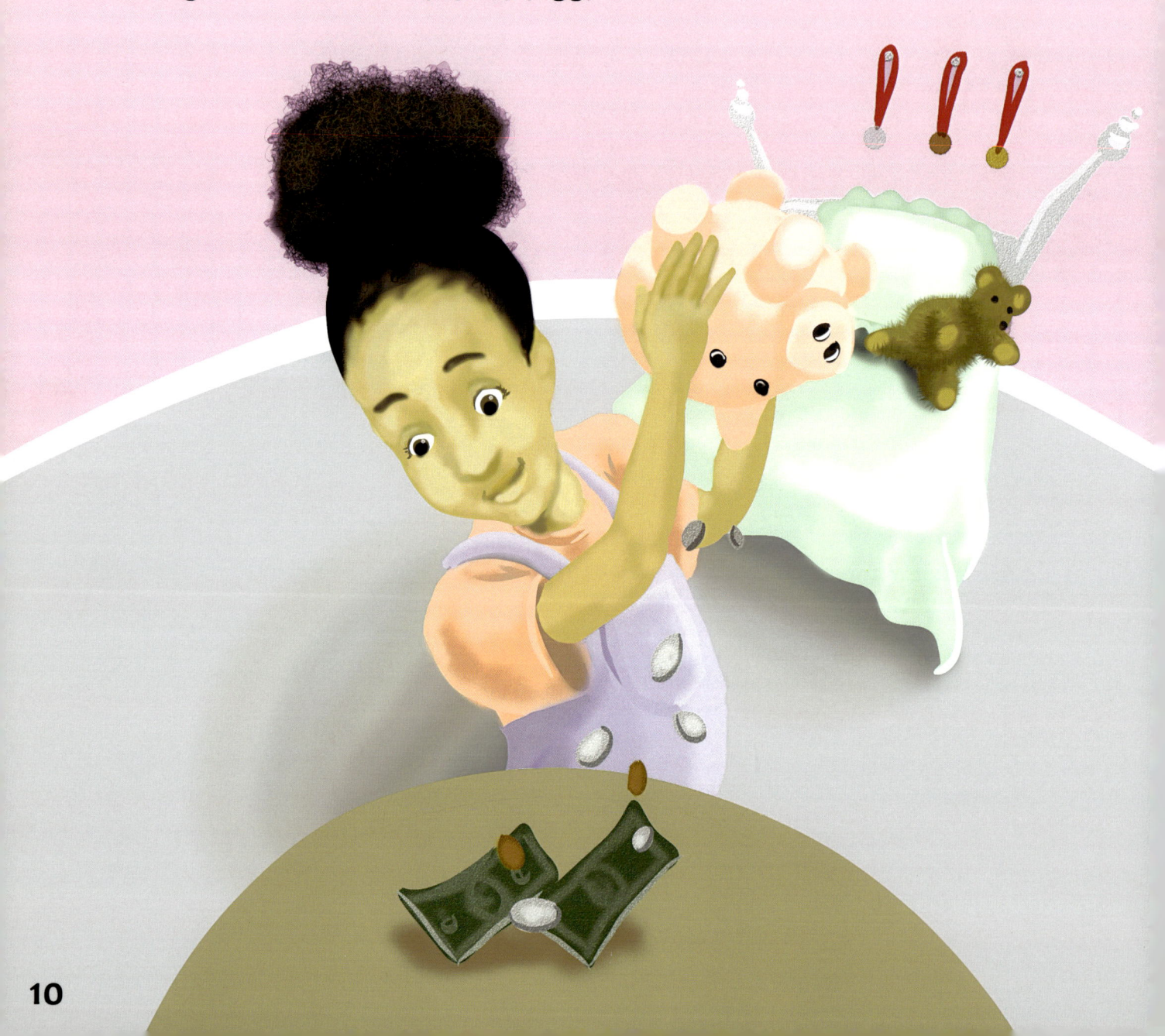

Returning home from a trip to the mall with Mom the next evening, a strange smell whizzes up my nose.

"NANA," I yell as I enter the kitchen, forgetting to use my inside voice. "Do you feel better?"

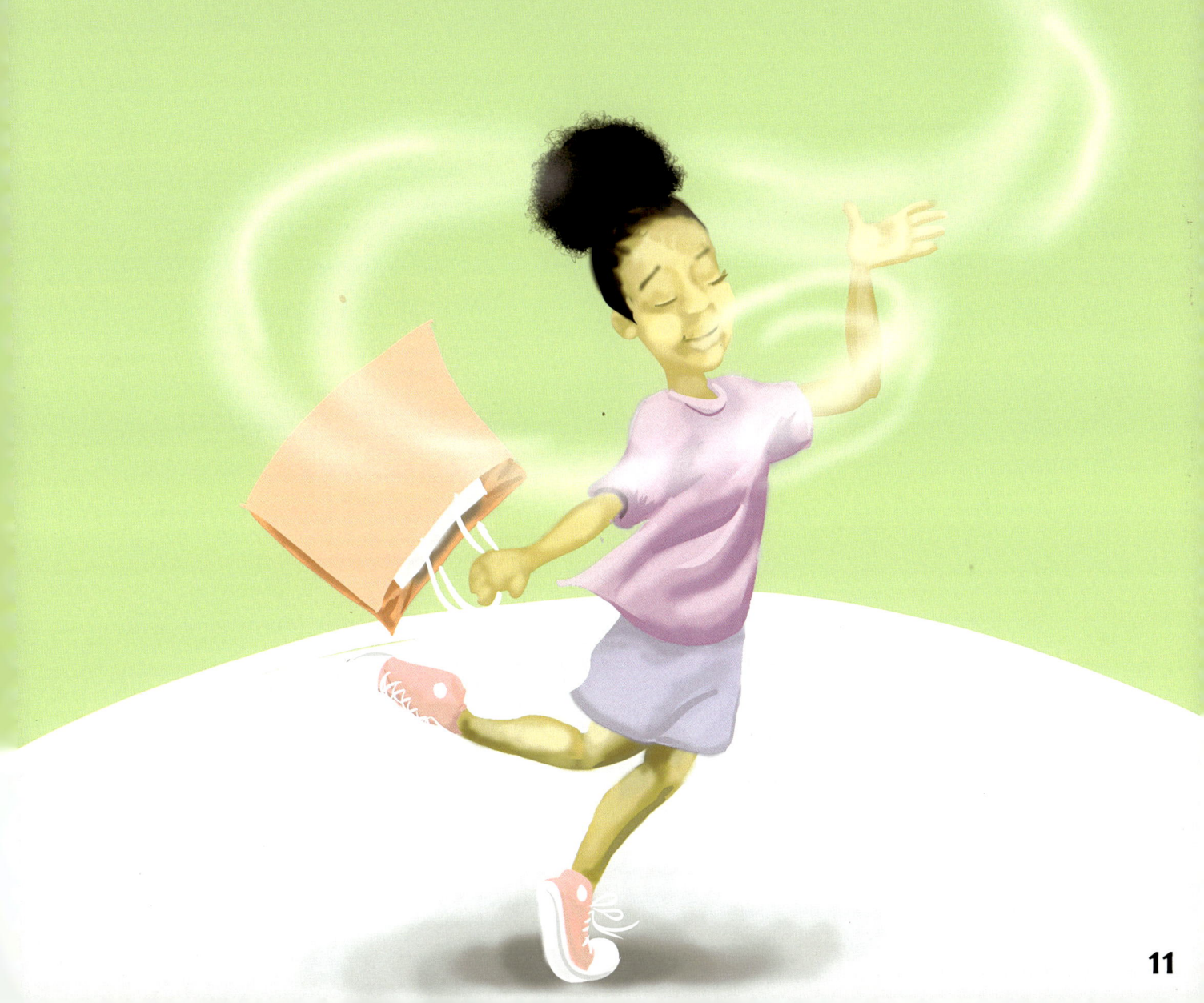

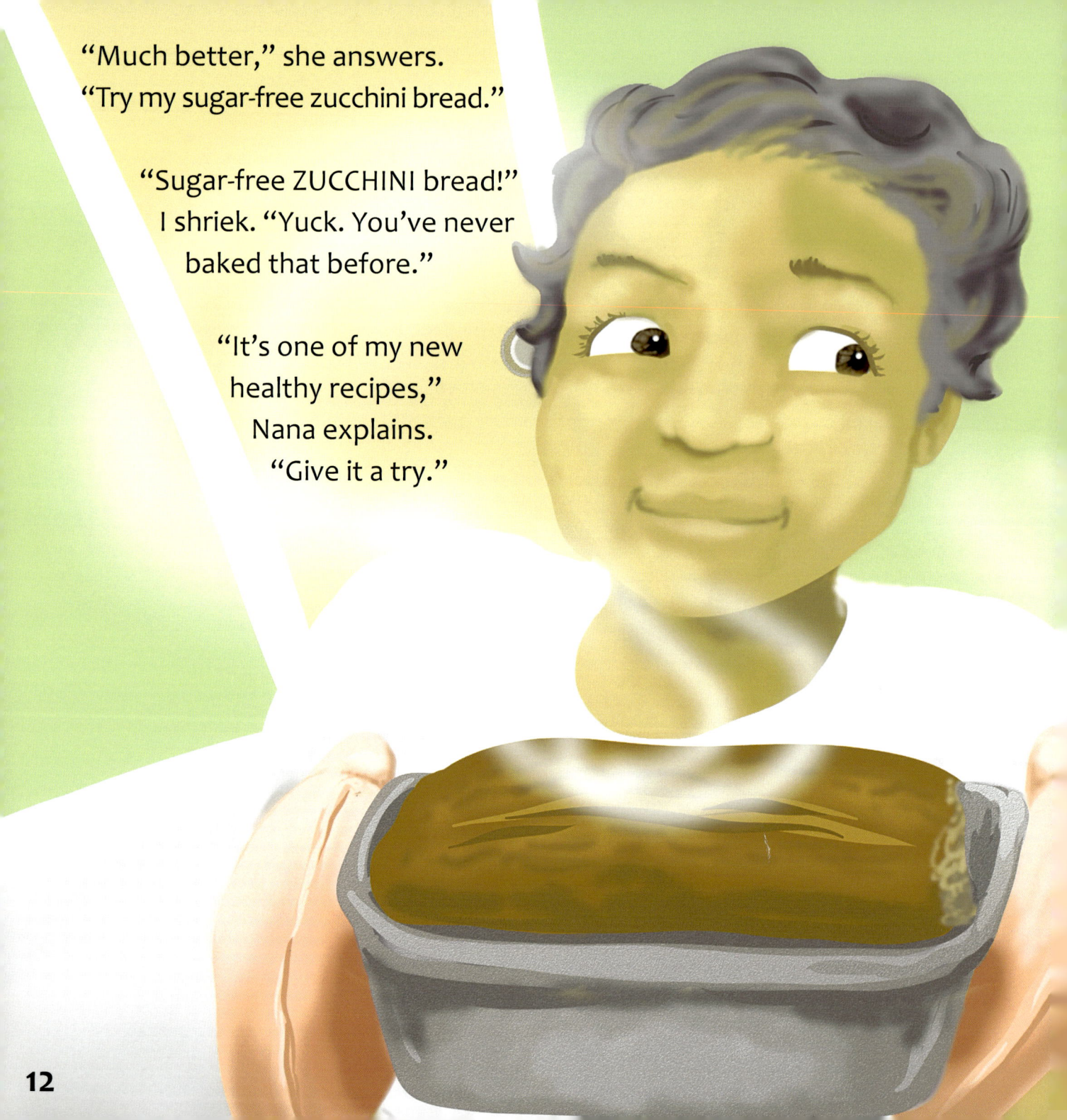

"Much better," she answers. "Try my sugar-free zucchini bread."

"Sugar-free ZUCCHINI bread!" I shriek. "Yuck. You've never baked that before."

"It's one of my new healthy recipes," Nana explains. "Give it a try."

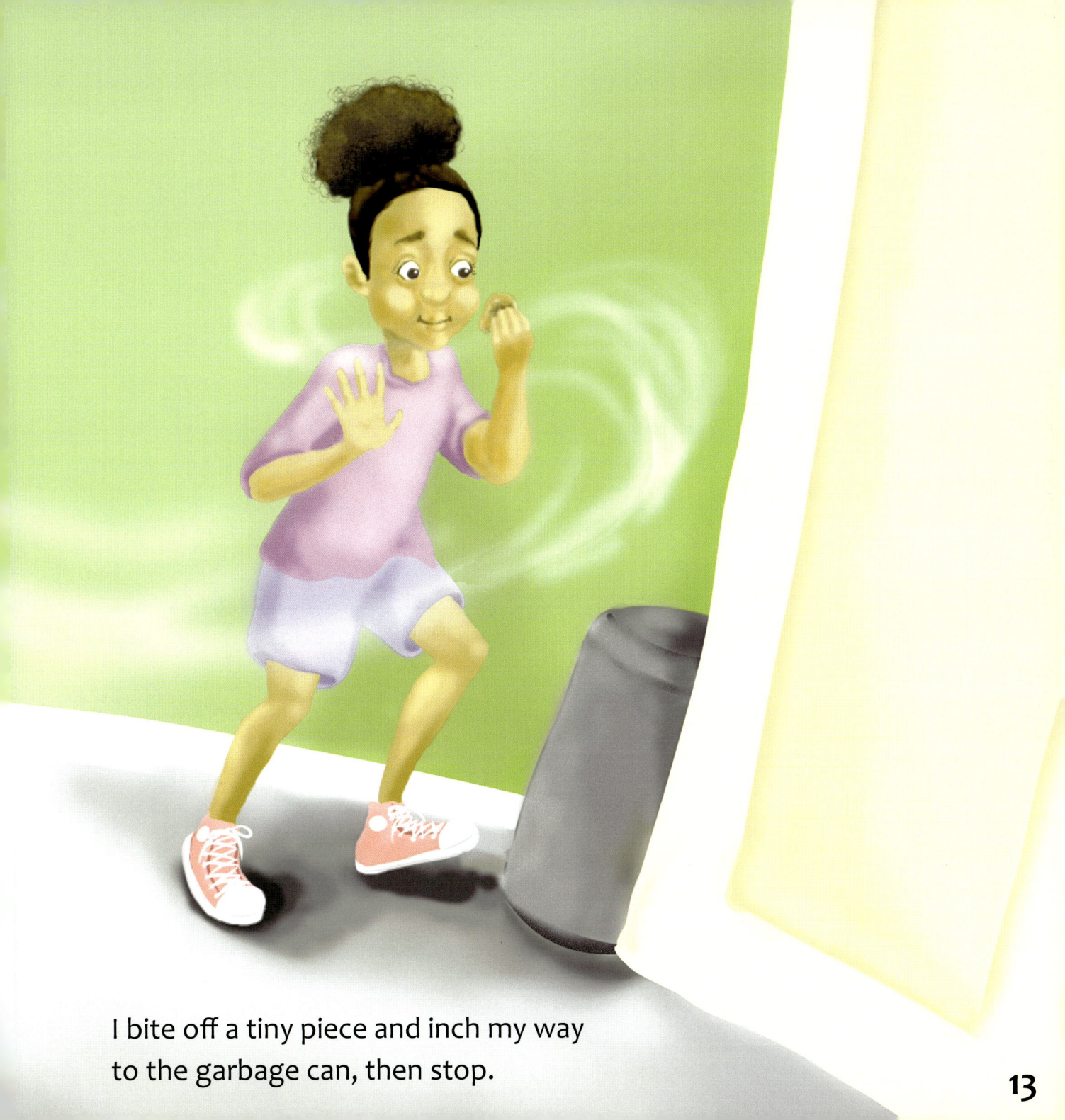

I bite off a tiny piece and inch my way to the garbage can, then stop.

13

14

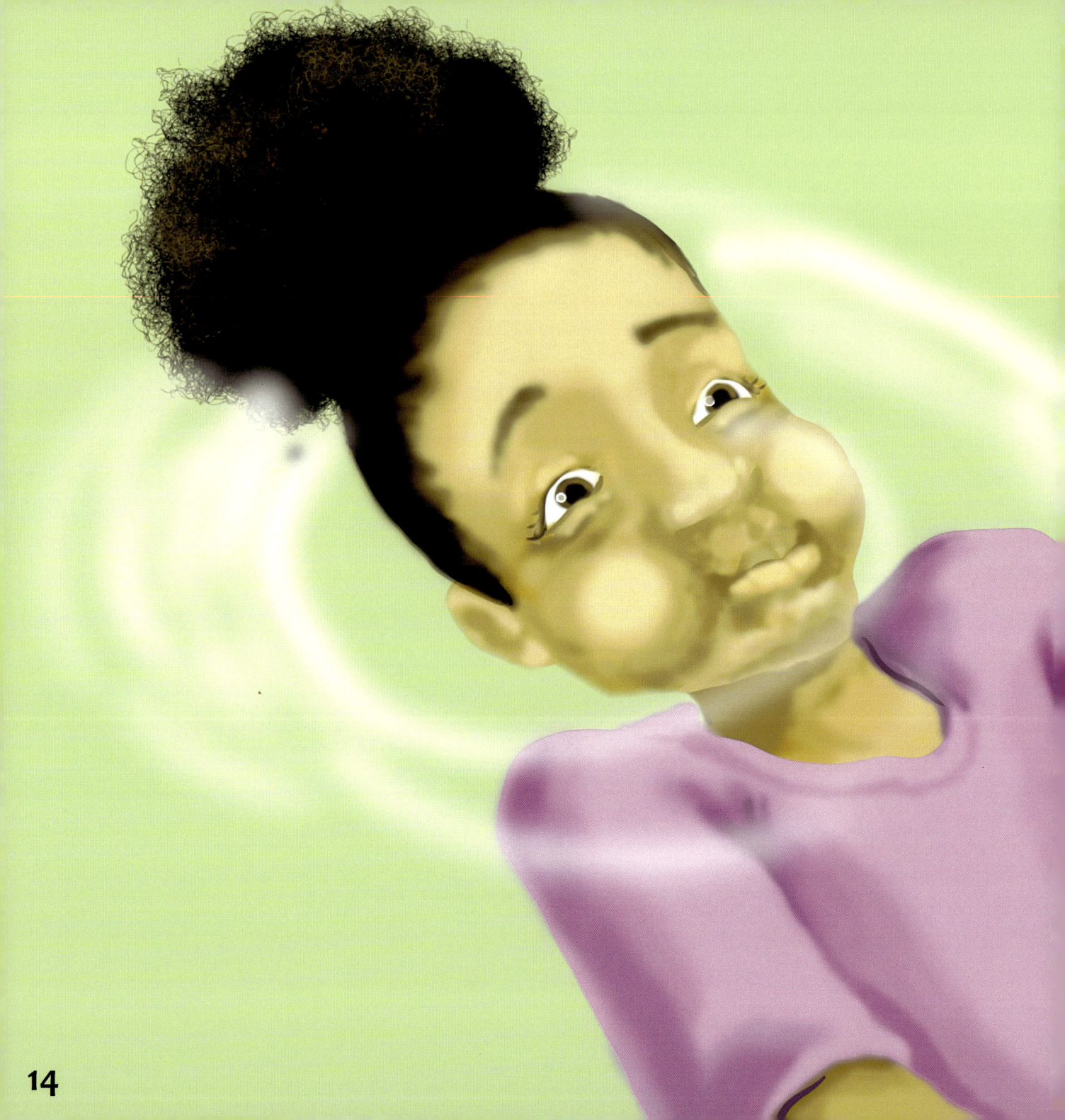

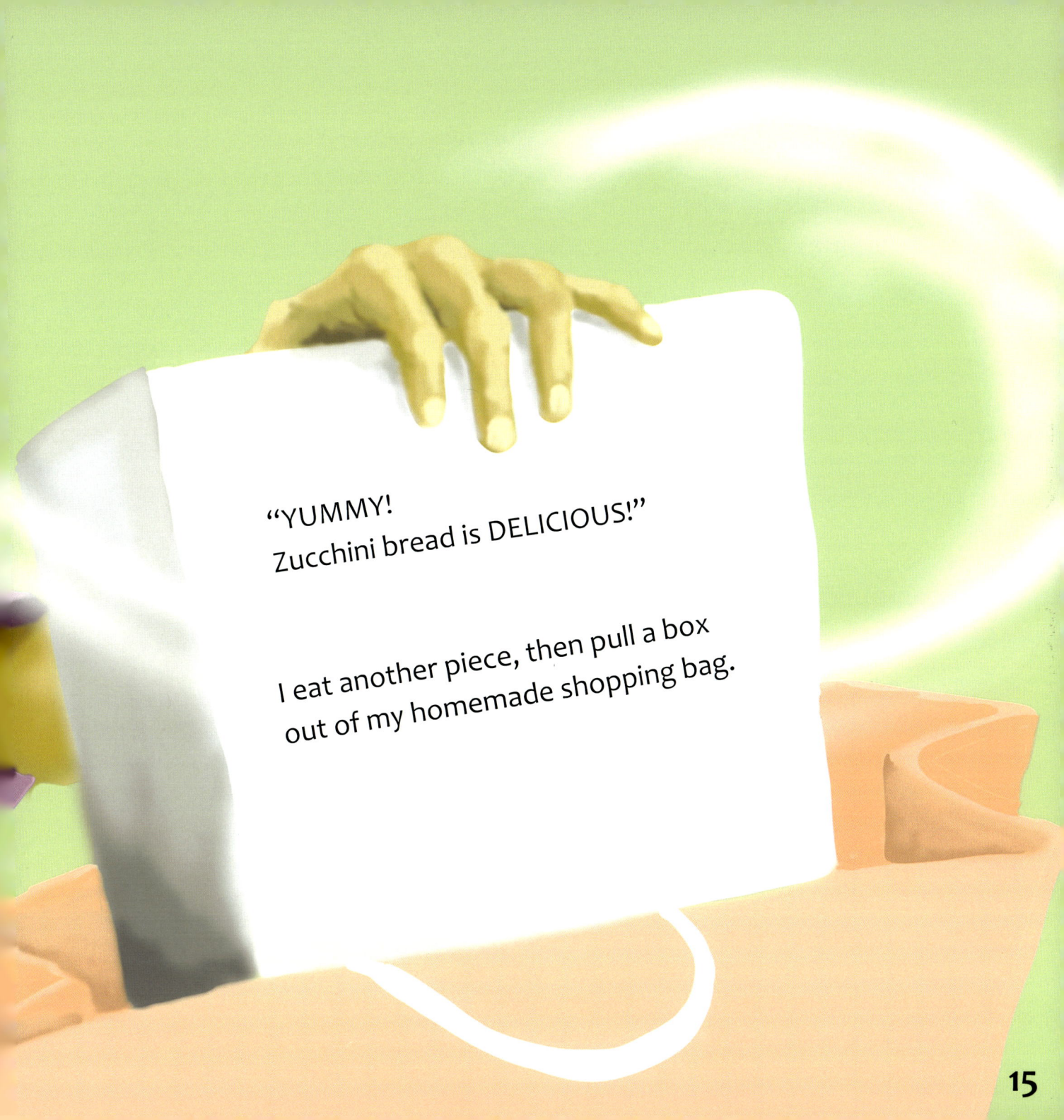

"YUMMY!
Zucchini bread is DELICIOUS!"

I eat another piece, then pull a box out of my homemade shopping bag.

"What is this?" Nana asks when I hand her the box.

"A special gift for you."

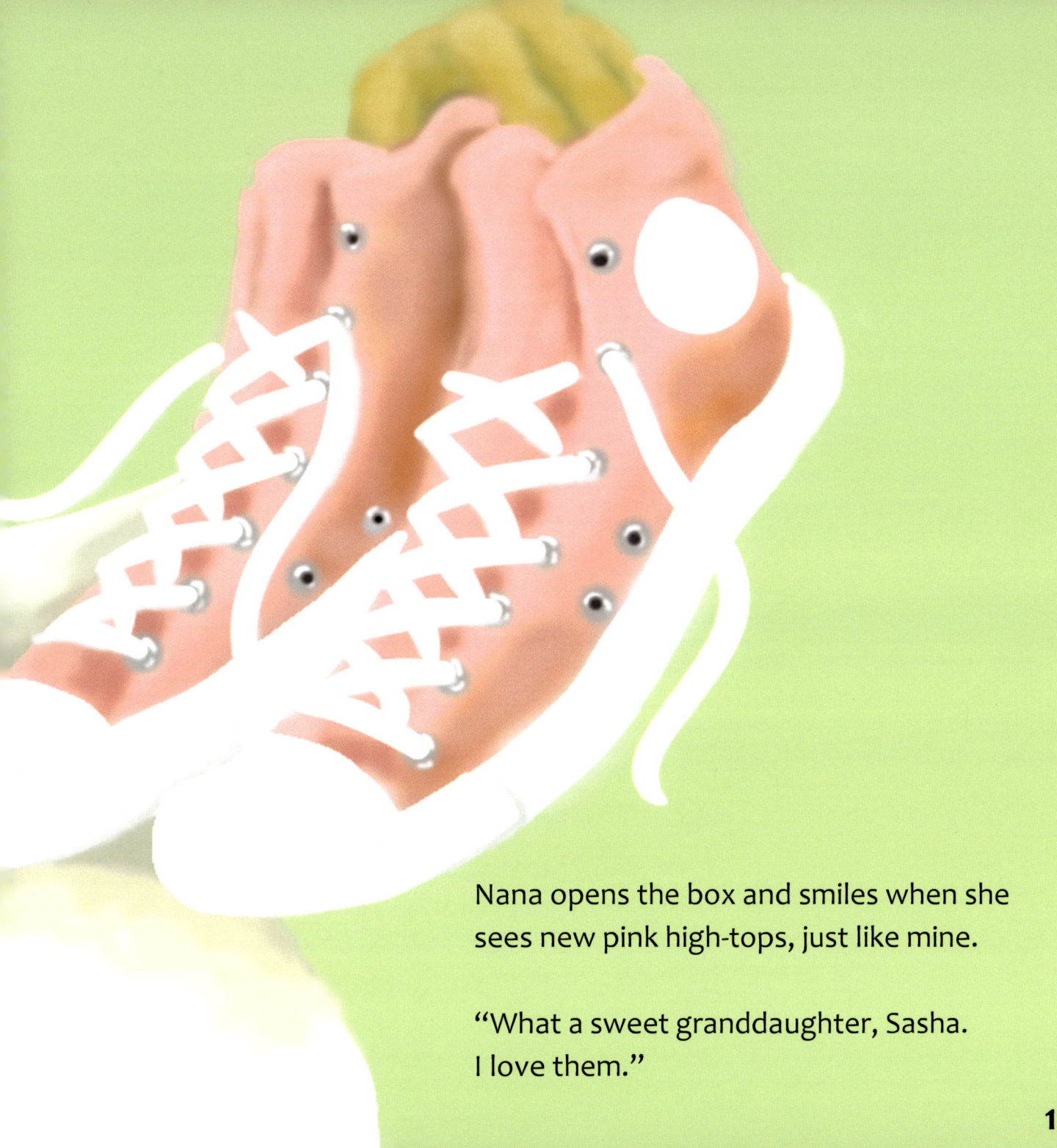

Nana opens the box and smiles when she sees new pink high-tops, just like mine.

"What a sweet granddaughter, Sasha. I love them."

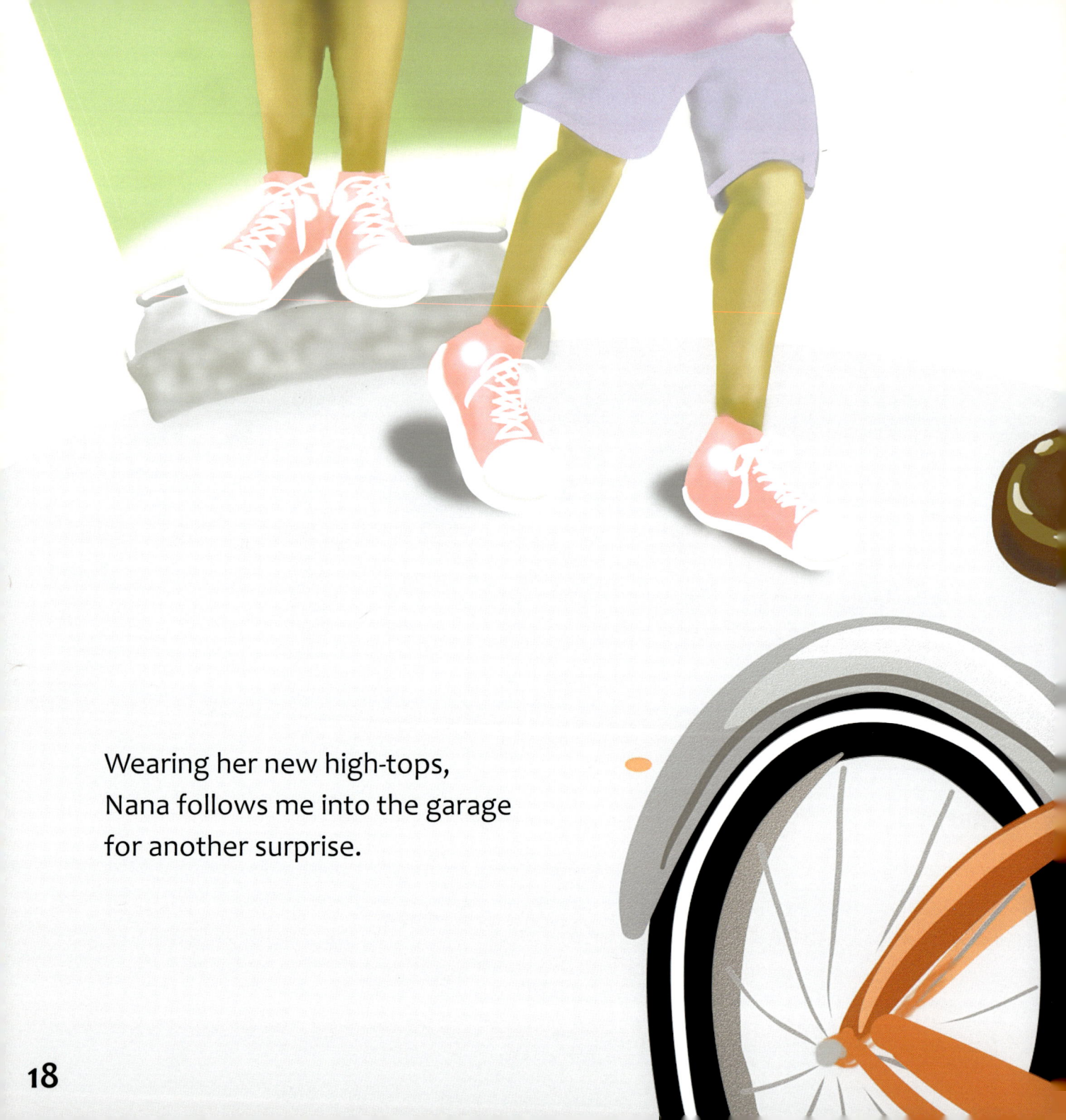

Wearing her new high-tops,
Nana follows me into the garage
for another surprise.

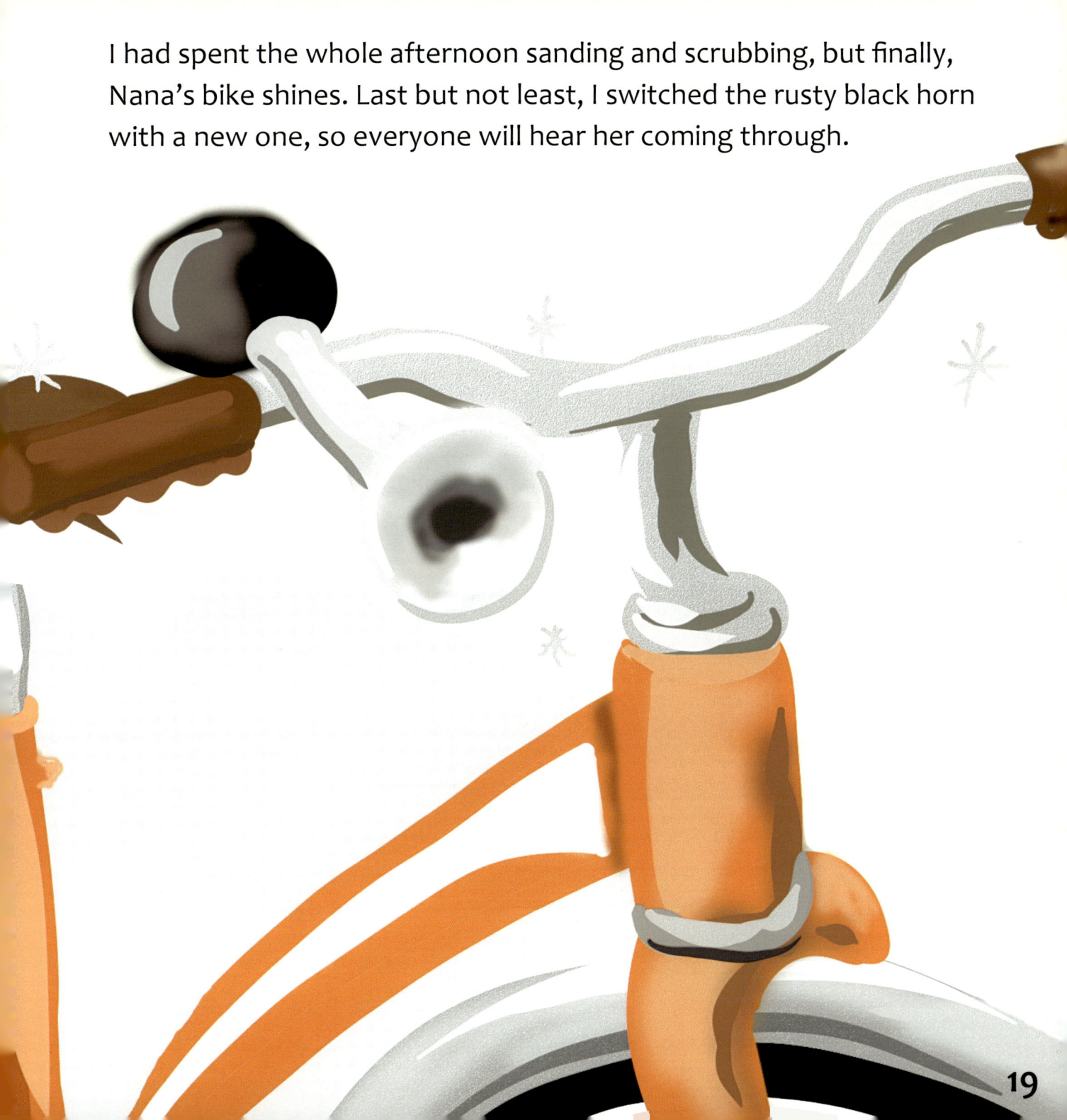

I had spent the whole afternoon sanding and scrubbing, but finally, Nana's bike shines. Last but not least, I switched the rusty black horn with a new one, so everyone will hear her coming through.

"Are you ready to ride?" I ask.

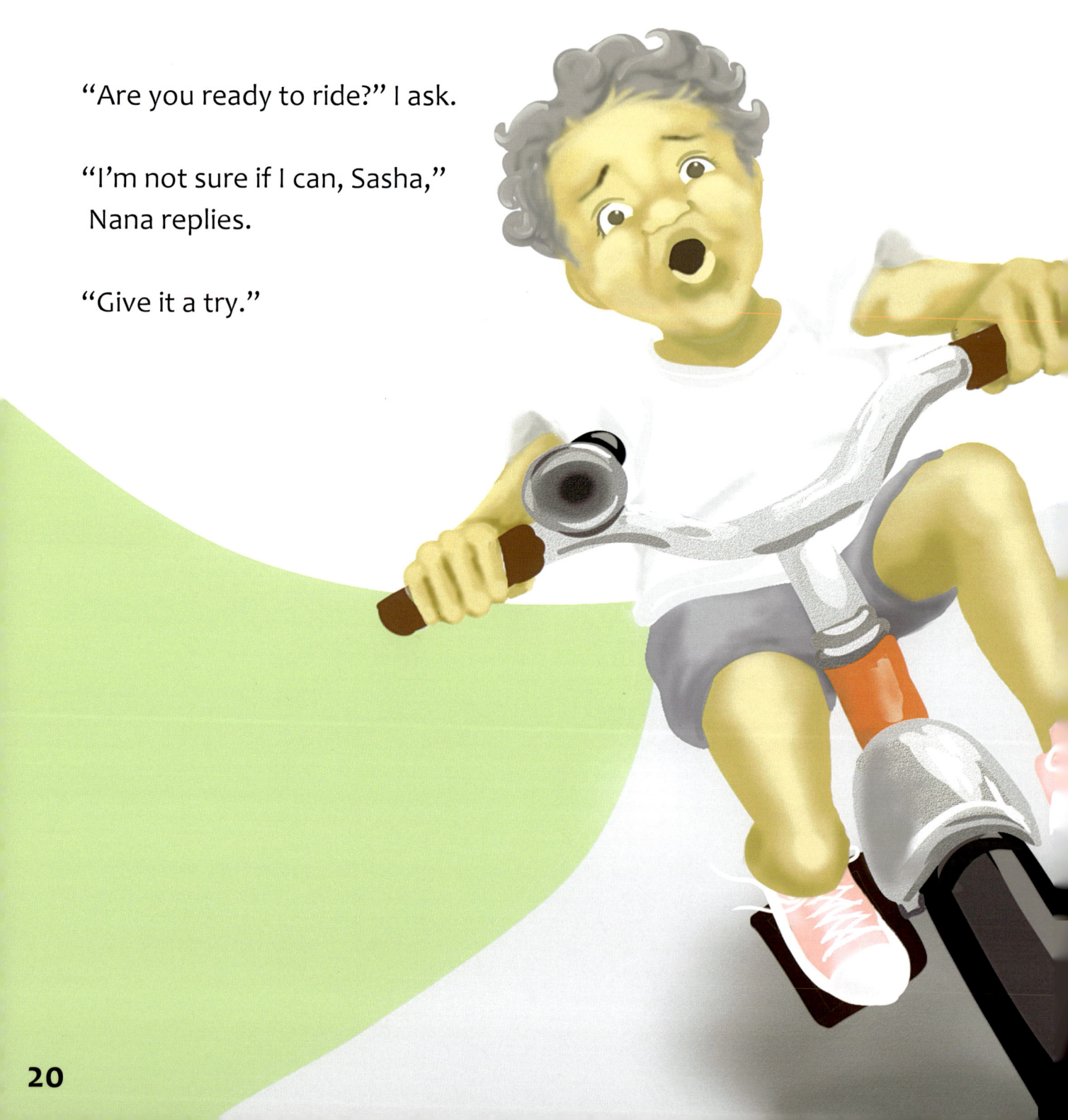

"I'm not sure if I can, Sasha," Nana replies.

"Give it a try."

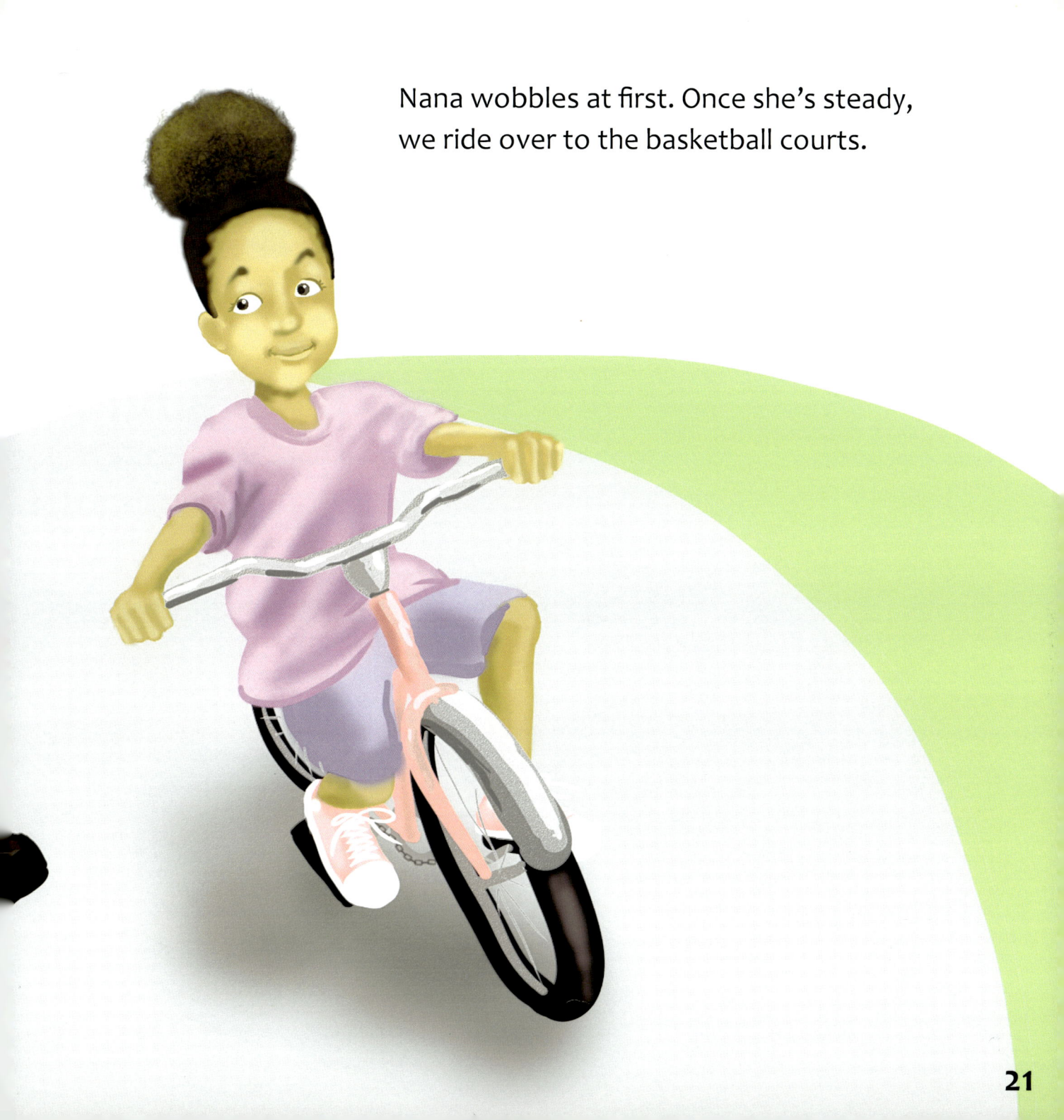

Nana wobbles at first. Once she's steady, we ride over to the basketball courts.

"Bet we can take on those boys for some hoops!"

Donning our matching pink high-tops, we play some fun 2-on-2.

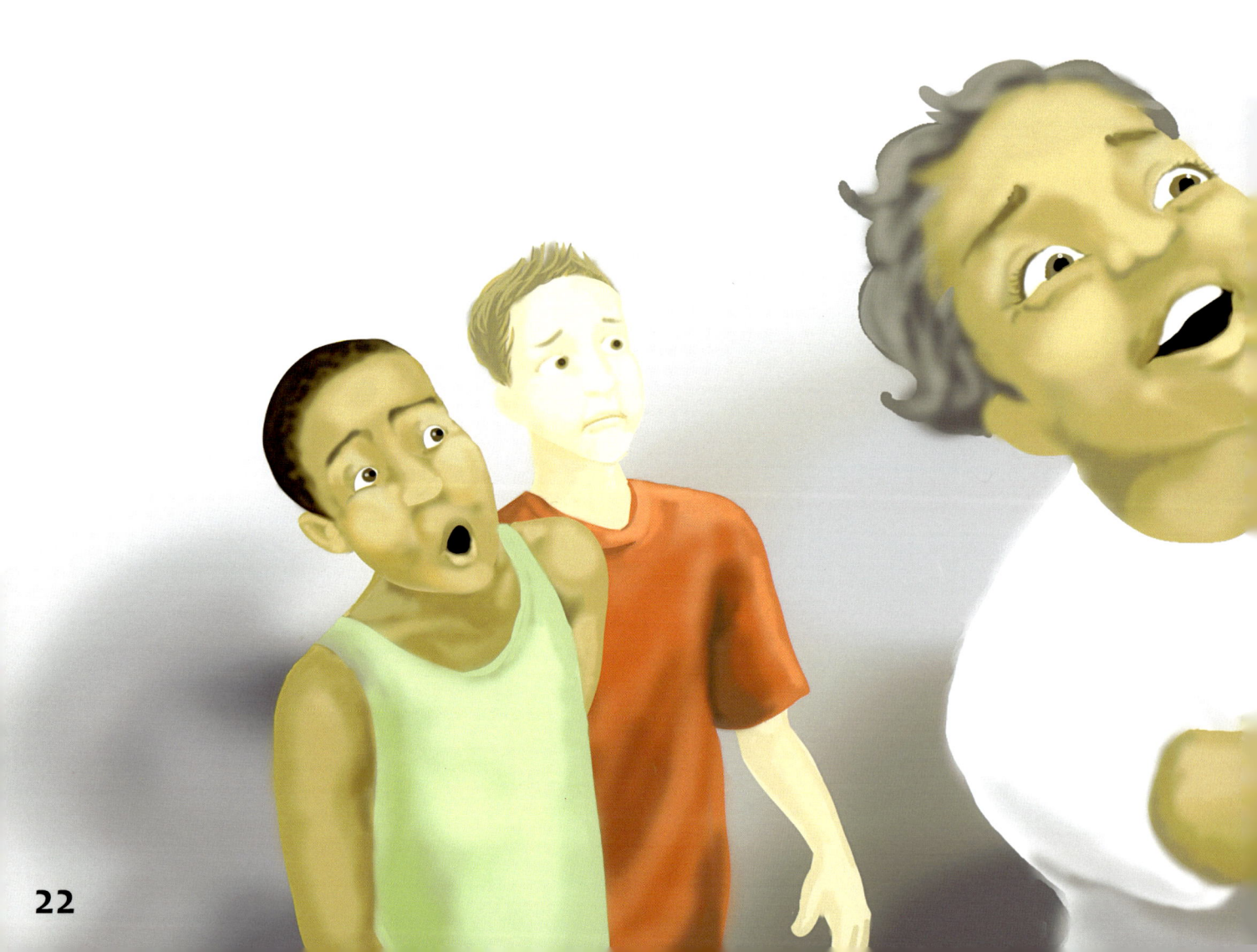

From that day on, zucchini bread became my favorite treat.

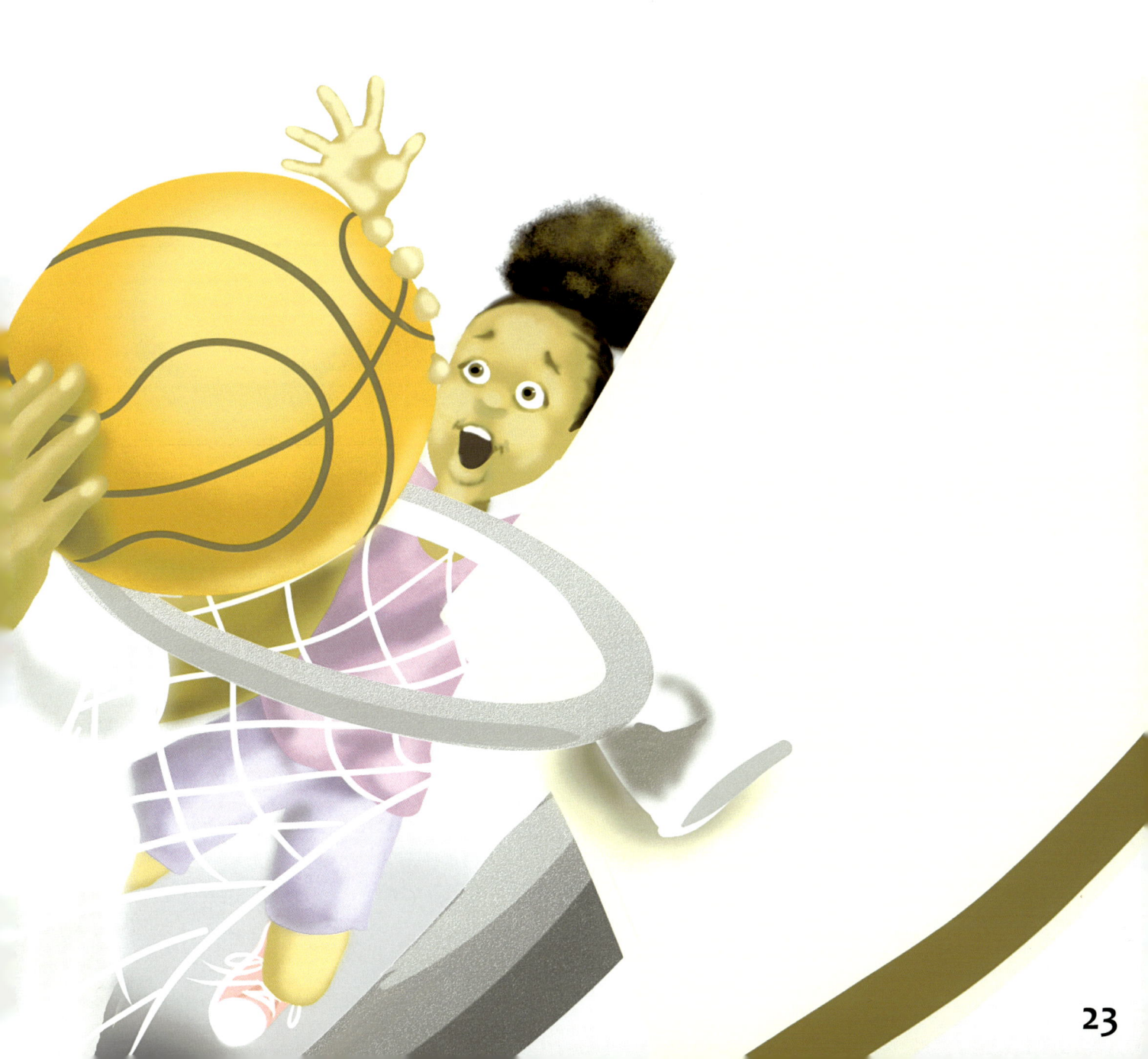

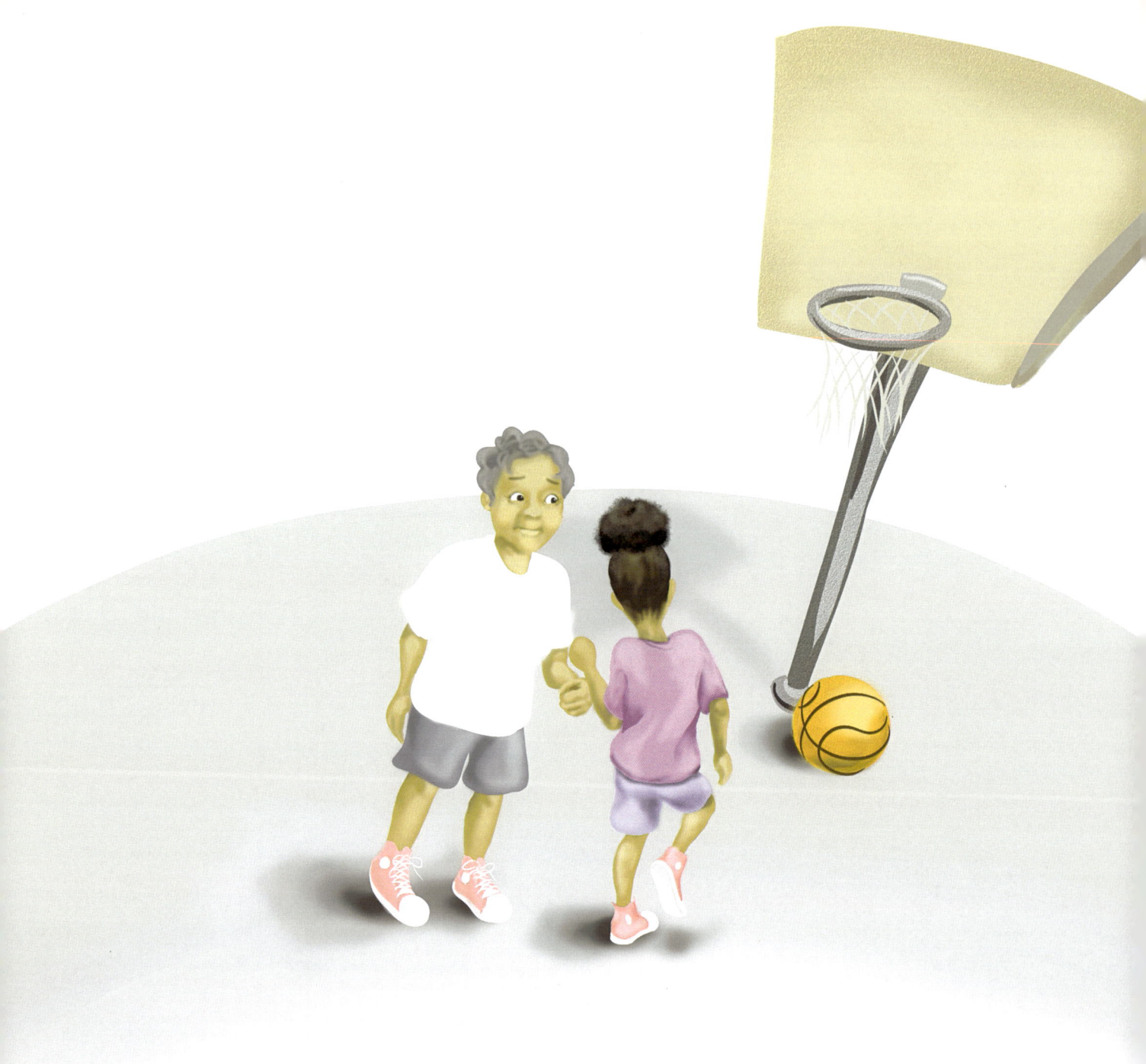

Shooting hoops and riding bikes became Nana's favorite things, too.

THE END

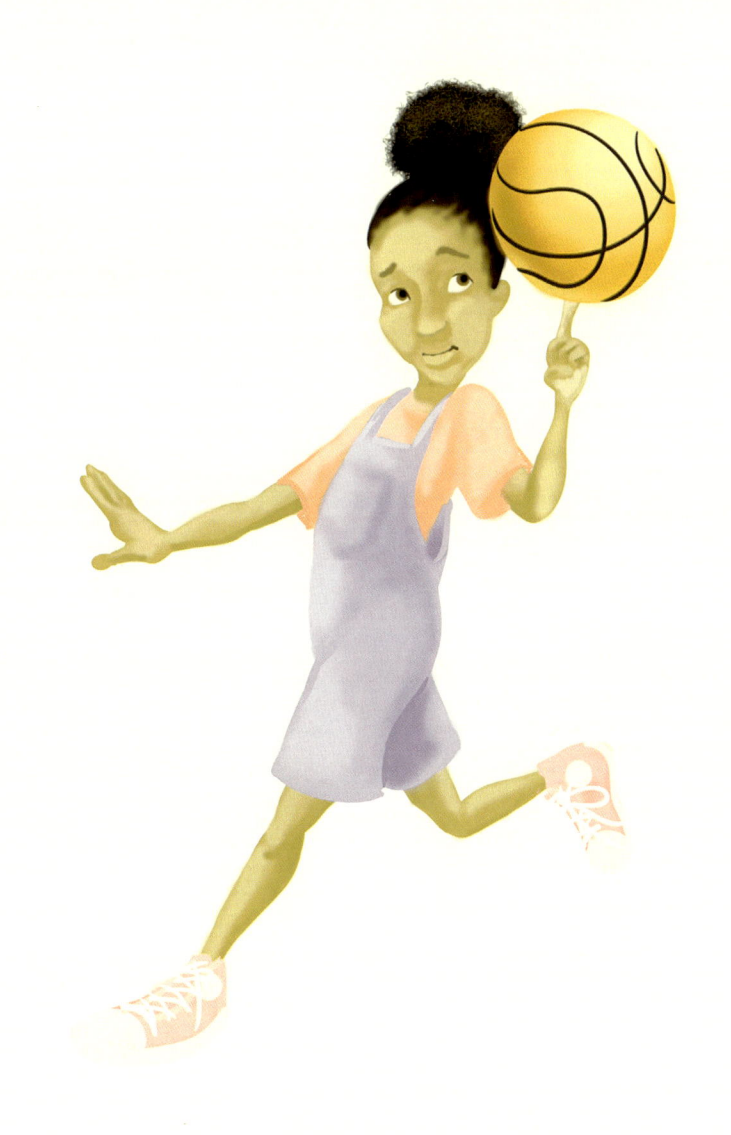

Nana's Zucchini Bread Recipe

Ingredients:

1 1/2 cup whole wheat pastry flour
1/2 teaspoon salt
1/2 teaspoon baking soda
1/2 teaspoon baking powder
1 teaspoon ground cinnamon
1/2 teaspoon ground nutmeg
2 eggs
1/3 cup unsweetened applesauce
2 tablespoons oil
1 cup vanilla yogurt
1 cup grated zucchini (remove excess water)
 1/3 cup chocolate (or carob) chips
(for a hint of sweetness)

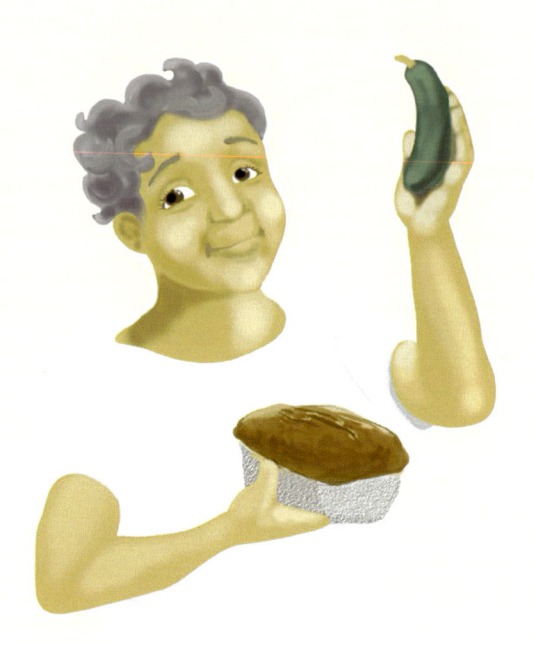

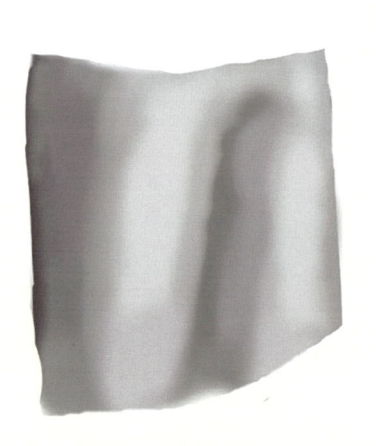

Steps:
- Preheat oven to 350°F. Spray an 8-inch loaf pan with natural cooking spray and set aside.
- Sift the dry ingredients into a large bowl (flour, salt, baking soda, baking powder, cinnamon and nutmeg)
- In a separate bowl, whisk together the eggs, yogurt, oil and applesauce.
- Add to flour mixture and stir until well combined.
- Fold in zucchini and walnuts (or alternatively, oats).
- Then pour batter into 2 pans and bake about 55 minutes (done when a toothpick comes out clean).
- Cool in pans on rack, then remove bread from pans.
- Enjoy!

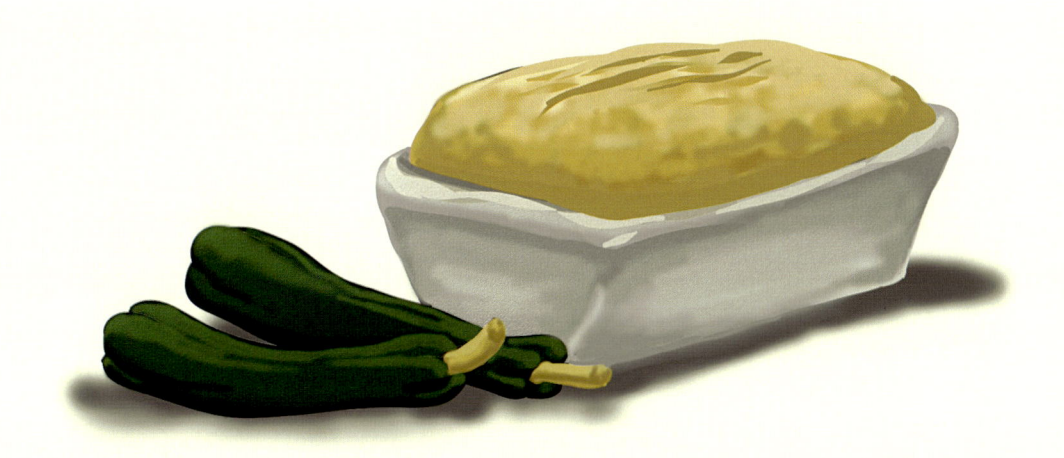

*For my family, Penny, TeMika,
and everyone who believed in my dream.*
D. H. P.

About the Author and Illustrator

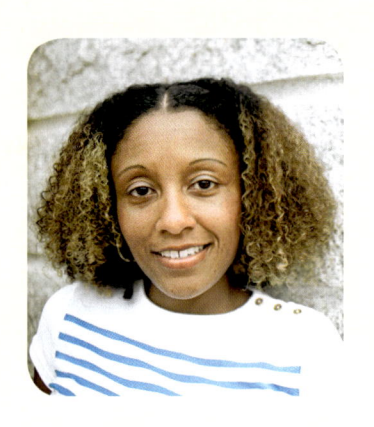

Dorothy H. Price *is a former high school English teacher. She enjoys teaching children fun and imaginative ways to write creatively through her Charlotte-based Young Authors Program.*

Diabetes has affected many of Dorothy's close relatives and friends. She is hopeful that Nana's Favorite Things will create dialogue around diabetes awareness and prevention. This is her first book.

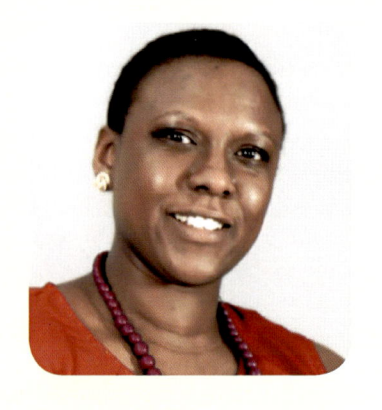

TeMika Grooms *is a visual artist and arts advocate who is inspired by great stories and the characters who live in them. She is intrigued by sequential art, specifically in the form of Children's Literature and Graphic Novels, as she recognizes herself as being a reluctant reader and visual learner early in life. TeMika uses her joy of learning through pictures as a way to teach and engage others in visual art and storytelling. She has presented workshops that encourages others to be creative, imaginative and gain freedom through story creation.*